Handbook for Monitoring

pH

Your Potential for Health

Dr. M. T. Morter, Jr.

IMPORTANT INFORMATION FOR THE READER

The information presented in this handbook has been compiled from my clinical experience and literary research. It is offered as a view of the relationship between food and health. This handbook is not a vehicle for, nor is it intended for, self-diagnosis or treatment of disease, nor is it a substitute for the advice and care of a licensed health care provider. This handbook is intended solely to help you make better judgements concerning your long-term health goals, and is not intended for the treatment of specific illnesses. No guarantee or assurance is given to anyone as to the specific results that may be obtained. If you are experiencing health problems, you should consult your doctor immediately. Remember, early examination and detection are important to successful treatment of all diseases.

ISBN# 0-944994-14-8

1000 West Poplar
Rogers, Arkansas 72756
(501) 631-2749
(800) 874-1478

CONTENTS

pH - YOUR POTENTIAL FOR HEALTH

Personal responsibility for personal health. That's the 21st century way. Proactive for health rather than reactive to disease. Disease is painful, activity-limiting, and costly. That's why checking personal pH – the acidity or alkalinity of some easy-to-get-to body fluids – will become as routine as checking your weight, credit card balance, or smoke alarm. Why? Because it can help you be an active participant in your personal health process. Keeping tabs on your personal pH can help you keep tabs on your personal health.

This pH handbook explains how to check the pH of readily accessible body fluids and interpret the results. It also gives a brief overview of what we might call "The Scope and Limitations" of pH monitoring. Knowing what you can't expect is as important as knowing what you can. And, perhaps most important, you will see how monitoring pH can help you be a more effective active participant in your personal pursuit of health.

This handbook is about evaluating your potential for health. It's not about diagnosing or curing disease. It's about monitoring signs of your body's ability to handle your diet and lifestyle. Diagnosing and curing are reactive. Monitoring is proactive. We are accustomed to focusing on disease care. Our usual perspective on health is to wait for disease to "strike," then try to combat it. Here we're presenting a different perspective – health. Rather than identifying a disease to fight, the objective is to find out if your diet and lifestyle are giving your body a fighting chance to be healthy.

This perspective on health is new to a lot of people. It's not the perspective of most of the medical community. Most health care is designed to help people control symptoms in order to "get better" or "feel better." Our objective here is to help you understand how you can "be better." The concepts and procedures presented here have developed over my thirty-plus years of clinical practice. They are not universally accepted by those whose job it is to diagnose, evaluate, and treat disease. However, the concepts presented here are a cornerstone for monitoring your health. Your health is your responsibility.

For too many years, we, as a nation, have had a tendency to leave the responsibility of our health to others. The general attitude has been, "I'll just do what I want and let the doctor fix it if something goes wrong." Our health care has been remedial. We wait until a problem crops up, then try to remedy it. We have proved that this system doesn't work. It's too painful for our bodies, too disruptive to our lifestyles, and too hard on our personal and national wallets. So, with the dawning of a new century, we also have the dawning of greater personal responsibility for our own health. Part of that responsibility is fulfilled by following the current trend of reducing fat intake and increasing the amount of fruits and vegetables we eat.

You have probably already taken steps to improve your diet. You probably eat foods that are lower in fat, cholesterol, and sodium than you used to. Another step is to adopt a habit of regular self-administered pH checks to see if your health improves along with your diet. Keeping track of how your body is withstanding your diet and lifestyle can be a major part of your newfound freedom that comes with taking personal responsibility for your personal health.

Notice that we are talking about keeping track of your health. We're not talking about diagnosing or treating. The concepts presented here are not intended to be used as a substitute for competent professional health care. They are to help you recognize clues that your body is being overstressed by your diet and lifestyle. Part of your responsibility for your health is to seek good professional care when you need it.

So, we'll begin with the basics of the what's and why's of pH, then move into the how-to and what-does-it-all mean.

WHAT IS pH?

In the scientific world, pH stands for "potential of Hydrogen." Or, you could be really scientific about it and say that pH represents the negative logarithm of the hydrogen ion concentration. Instead, for purposes for this book, we'll just say that, in your body, pH stands for your potential for Health.

pH is the value given to indicate the acidity or alkalinity of a substance. It's a value – an intangible, not a thing. You can't pick it up, use it to buy a jet ski, or dip it in your soup. pH values are to acid and alkaline what temperature degrees are to heat and cold.

The pH scale of values runs from 0 to 14. At the low end, 0 indicates really strong, complete acidity. At the high end, 14 indicates really strong, complete alkalinity. In the middle, pH 7.0 indicates that the substance is neither acid nor alkaline – it's neutral. Very few substances are completely neutral. Most substances test out on either side of neutral. The pH of most substances falls somewhere from very strong to very weak acid, or from very weak to very strong alkali. For example, at pH 2.5, vinegar is a strong acid, and at pH 8.0, baking soda is mildly (that's more than "slightly") alkaline. But we're not concerned with vinegar or baking soda here. We're talking body fluids. We're concerned with the pH of your "internal environment" – the potential for Health of the fluids in and around your cells. When we talk about the pH of your body, we mean the pH of the fluids inside and outside your cells.

BODY CHECK

To find out how the pH of your internal fluids are faring, specially treated test paper is used to check some of the fluids your body generates. pH test paper is designed specifically to indicate pH values. The paper you'll use registers pH values, essentially in two-tenths increments, from moderately strong acid of pH 5.5 to mildly alkaline pH 8.0. The thin strip of pH paper changes color when it comes in contact with moist or wet acid or alkaline substances. A color guide comes with the pH paper dispenser. This guide shows the colors the paper can register. Each color represents a particular pH value. The numerical value is shown above each color sample.

So that's the test equipment you'll use – pH paper. And what do you use it on?

Even though your blood is the most important fluid in your body, you don't "open a vein" to check your internal pH. Tears and perspiration take effort to generate, so they're out. Other more readily available fluids are urine and saliva. The details of the checking procedure are given later. For now, you need to understand what you are trying to accomplish by checking the pH of either urine or saliva.

The purpose of checking urine pH is to find out if your body has a healthy store of the minerals that keep its internal environment slightly alkaline. Alkalizing minerals neutralize, or counteract, strong acid. Another term for the neutralizing process that means essentially the same thing is "buffering." In other words, alkalizing minerals make strong acid weaker, or not acid at all. This store of alkalizing minerals is your alkaline reserve – the workhorse of a very important buffer system. The minerals that contribute to your alkaline reserve are sodium, calcium, potassium, magnesium, and iron. Your alkaline reserve isn't a single cubby hole within your body where these important minerals loll around waiting to be summoned. Your alkaline reserve is scattered throughout your body in various organs.

Urine pH values are your clue to whether or not your alkaline arsenal has been, or is being, used up or overwhelmed. The pH values indicate whether or not your body is overburdened with too much acid from too much high protein food. Saliva pH values, on the other hand, are your guide to whether or not your body is overburdened with emotional stress.

Urine pH and saliva pH results are valid only if checked under controlled conditions. That is, you set the scene first. Random or willy-nilly checks of the pH of either of these fluids may be interesting, but they're meaningless. With a little planning before you whip our your pH paper, you get something to hang your health on.

As a preview of coming instructions, you set the scene for checking your urine pH by eating particular types of foods for two days immediately before the big check. To prepare for your saliva pH test, don't eat, drink, chew gum, suck on a cough drop, or put anything else in your mouth except water for at least two hours.

pH AND HEALTH

Monitoring your pH gives you an indication of how well or how hard your body is working to survive your lifestyle. Notice that I said "it gives you an *indication* . . ." The results of your pH tests are *indicators* of how your body is responding to the foods you eat and to other stresses. The actual acid or alkaline level of your internal environment affects how your body functions. The pH values you get when you test your urine or saliva are indications of how your body is functioning.

When your body is at its pH best, it hums along smoothly and easily. When your body hums along smoothly and easily, your life has a good chance of doing the same. When your body is at less than its pH best, its hum may turn into an exhausted moan as it works overtime to survive. And, when your body is exhausted, you are exhausted.

The pH of your internal environment is a good indicator of how hard your body is working just to survive. The ideal pH for most of the fluids of your internal environment is just above pH 7.0. That's slightly alkaline. Your body functions best when the pH of most of its fluids hover in the pH 7.0 neighborhood. Your blood must be a slightly alkaline pH 7.35 to pH 7.45 all the time. That's a "must," not an "it-would-be-nice." If the pH of your blood falls much below 7.35 or rises much above 7.45 for more than a few hours, you can't survive. When your other bodily fluid pH values are too far below or too high above pH 7.0, your potential for health plummets.

Although your blood is slightly alkaline, the fluids in your stomach are usually quite acid. Digestive fluids may be as low as pH 1.0. That's strong acid. This strong acid helps to "break down" the foods you eat as they begin their journey through your body. When we talk about the pH of the body, we're not talking about stomach pH. We're talking about the fluid in and around your cells.

CHECKING pH IS NOT A DIAGNOSTIC TEST

As a rule, we go to a doctor when we have a specific pain, problem, or symptom. Rarely does a doctor hear the complaint, "I'm feeling great. Fix it." Our health focus is usually on identifying symptoms and trying to get rid of them. When a doctor orders lab tests for you, these tests are to find out if a problem exists in a particular organ or system. We concentrate on identifying parts of the body that are the source of our misery. Not so with a pH check.

Monitoring your pH helps you *evaluate* how your *whole body* is doing. It's a health index evaluation process, not a disease identifying process. Your pH doesn't tell you whether or not you have a life-impairing, or life-threatening disease. You can't look at your pH results and correctly conclude, "Mercy me, I have galloping graphospasm!" **pH tests don't diagnose!**

Your pH checks are not diagnostic tests. They are evidence to use in evaluating your overall health. Your internal pH concerns your whole body. Not parts. Knowing the pH of your body won't tell you if your liver is functioning perfectly. It won't tell you if your pancreas is struggling to produce insulin. It won't tell you if your blood pressure is running amuck. It won't tell you if you are anemic or overweight or nearsighted. Checking your pH is not a diagnostic test. **This cannot be emphasized too strongly**.

If you find that your internal pH is higher or lower than "ideal," you won't know any more than you did before about which, if any, disease you may have. However, you will have a strong indication that your body's systems and organs are working under extreme stress of toxicity – its internal fluids are being "poisoned" by too much acid. But that doesn't mean you have a particular disease. It means that unless you change your ways (probably starting with the types of food you eat), you *could* develop a disease. Remember, pH is an indicator of the condition of your internal environment. And, your internal environment affects your overall health.

Perhaps a disease label has already been attached to your symptoms. If so, the chances that your organs and systems are living in an ideal pH neighborhood are about as good as your chances of being the first person to hit a golf ball on Jupiter. Knowing the pH value of your internal environment won't cure your disease any more than knowing your blood pressure will cure hypertension. However, it can give you a clue that your body is "fighting stress" rather than "fighting disease." The disease is an effect of the stress of your body coping in a "tough neighborhood."

THERE GOES THE NEIGHBORHOOD

Some types of foods you eat can mess up your internal environment. They leave an acid "mess" that the body must neutralize and eliminate. These messy foods are essentially high-protein foods – meats, poultry, fish, and grains. They are acid ash-producing foods. Most of us eat a lot of acid ash foods. That's our custom, tradition, and a large part of our economy. But acid ash foods leave the internal equivalent of blowing trash, beer cans, drug paraphernalia, derelict cars, and graffiti. In other words, junk! Messy junk that pollutes the internal area and environment.

The "junk" from acid ash foods is in the form of an acid residue that's left after high-protein food has been digested. We might say it's the physiological equivalent of toxic waste. During digestion, the usable parts of food are absorbed to help nourish the body. But a residue that can't be used is left. This residue is acid. The body doesn't need it. The acid of this residue can be quite strong. The residue itself will eventually make its way through the kidneys or bowel and out of the body. However, before it is eliminated, it must be neutralized – weakened, buffered. If it isn't neutralized, it can fry delicate kidney tissue. That's not good.

However, our bodies are smarter than we will ever be. Your own smart body has all sorts of ways to protect itself. The primary protection against strong acid is alkalizing minerals. These vital minerals can neutralize, or tone down, the acid from "quite strong" to "slightly strong." Pretty clever. Unfortunately, in the process of neutralizing the acid, the minerals are eliminated right along with the residue. The vital neutralizing minerals tag along with the acid all the way out of your body. Gone forever. That's the bad news.

The good news is that these lost minerals are easily replaced. Replacements come from the fruits and vegetables you eat. No problem – acid in the body is neutralized by minerals, replacement minerals come along in fruits and vegetables to take their place.

But suppose you don't eat fruits and vegetables – well, not much, anyway.

Your intelligent body isn't going to let a little thing like your negligence keep it from doing what needs to be done. Your body is a survivor. It was designed to survive. It wasn't designed to be healthy or sick. If minerals that were lost aren't replaced, other minerals jump in to do the job – survival. But these substitute minerals weren't just sitting on the bench waiting to be called into the game. They have important full-time jobs, too. When they are called on to handle the emergency, they are taken from their primary jobs. For example, calcium is a "substitute" neutralizing mineral. Where do we keep our biggest calcium supply? Our bones. If you don't replace neutralizing minerals by eating fruits and vegetables, calcium is taken from the bones. You know what happens when you lose a lot of calcium from your bones. The disease label is "osteoporosis." The practical effect is weak bones. And it's hard to hold your head up when your spine is gradually collapsing.

Your diet can be so top-heavy with acid ash foods that your neutralizing, or buffering, systems are overwhelmed. There is just too much acid for them to handle – acid saturation. When acid laden materials arrive at the kidneys, the kidneys must act to neutralize the acid fast. It's another backup system. Ammonia. Your kidneys generate ammonia which has a pH of about 9.25. A little ammonia mixed with strong acid raises the pH value. A lot of ammonia in a strong acid raises the pH value a lot.

So when your body is too acid for too long, it plays the game of life with a lineup of backup systems. These backups are either substitute minerals, or ammonia. When your body is too acid – when your internal pH is too low – the systems and organs of your body work overtime just to stay even. But systems and organs aren't designed to function flat-out in red-alert mode all the time. They need rest just as you do. If the red-alert goes on for months or years, systems and organs become exhausted. An exhausted body can't compete with disease. Eventually, disease wins the game.

What does all of this have to do with checking pH?

Monitoring your pH periodically gives you a status report on the quality of the environment of your internal neighborhood. Remember, pH monitoring doesn't report on how the systems, organs, and processes are doing. It is your personal "neighborhood watch."

Of course, that's not a scientific explanation of how your physiological processes work. However, it may give you an idea of how the pH of your body affects your potential health and how the environment of a perfectly good internal neighborhood can be ruined. The process boils down to . . .

1. Acid ash from many of the foods you regularly eat must be neutralized (buffered) before the acid is eliminated through the kidneys.
2. Vital minerals are used to neutralize the acid, and in the process these minerals are lost through the kidneys and bowel.
3. If the neutralizing minerals aren't replaced, other minerals will be taken from other functions to neutralize the acid.
4. If the neutralizing (buffer) systems aren't up to the task, or if the body is saturated with acid, the kidneys generate ammonia as a last-ditch effort.
5. The body is over-acid, buffer systems are overwhelmed, and systems, organs, and processes are overstressed.
6. The body's systems and organs aren't able to perform at their best because they have become exhausted.

That's principally what you learn from checking your urine pH – whether or not the foods you eat regularly have exhausted your body's systems and organs.

MORE ACID

Your body works constantly to get rid of acid no matter where it comes from. Acid ash-producing food isn't the only source of acid in your body. Two other prominent sources contribute to your internal acid level: (1) cellular activity, and (2) naturally acid foods. First, self-generated acid from cellular activity.

Your cells produce acid as they function. As long as cells are alive, they work and produce acid. As cells die off, other cells replace them. The new cells also produce acid. So, as long as you are alive, new cells are being produced, and cells are producing acid. In addition, when you exercise, cells produce more acid than when you're resting. Acid production is a standard procedure for your body.

That's strange! The body works best when it is in a slightly alkaline environment. Staying alkaline is so important that the body uses and loses vital minerals as it gets rid of acid. Yet the body produces acid.

That's right. *Your body is alkaline by design and acid by function.*™ That is a very important concept. Alkaline by design; acid by function. However, there's a big difference between the acid your cells produce and the acid that you get in high-protein acid ash producing foods. In the first place, the acid from cells – physiological acid, it's called – is a lot weaker than acid from high-protein acid ash foods. And in the second place, self-produced cellular acid doesn't need to be neutralized by vital minerals before it is sent out of the body. Self-produced cellular acid is easily eliminated through your lungs when you breathe and when you talk.

You also get acid from foods, such as oranges and lemons, that are acid in their own right. This acid is also different from the acid you get from acid ash-producing foods. And, it is as easily eliminated as the acid cells produce. This concept gets a little tricky, so we'll clear it up a bit.

We have talked a lot about *acid ash-producing foods* that leave an acid residue after they get into the body. By now you know that acid ash foods are generally high – protein meats, poultry, fish, and grains. Now we're talking about *acid foods* that are acid when they go into the body. They are naturally acid. Lemons, oranges, and grapefruit are obviously acid. In fact, they are so acid that many people can't eat them without suffering discomfort. In general, fruits and vegetables are naturally acid foods.

In their natural state, acid foods – fruits and vegetables – have more built-in acid than do high protein acid ash-producing foods – meat, poultry, fish, and grains. Fruit acid especially may be fairly strong going into your body. However, your body can get rid of fruit and vegetable acid very easily. The tag-along acid from fruits and vegetables is eliminated the same way as the acid generated by your cells. You just blow it off.

The acid from acid ash-producing foods is different. This is the kind of acid that needs to be neutralized before it is eliminated from your body. You can't just blow it off. It must be weakened and escorted by neutralizing minerals out of the body through kidneys or bowel.

The acid of fruits and vegetables is no problem. The acid from ash of meats, poultry, fish, and grains can be a problem.

Just as high-protein foods leave a residual ash, fruits and vegetables also leave an ash residue. However, despite the naturally acid nature of fruits or vegetables, generally, the ash they leave is not acid. There's a big difference between the ash left by fruits and vegetables and the ash left by high-protein acid ash-producing foods. The ash left by most fruits and vegetables is alkaline. It contains minerals that help alkalize your body.

Fruits are pretty neat additions to your body. They're not big stress producers. They are easily digested. The acid that comes in them is easily eliminated through the lungs. And the ash they leave contributes needed minerals for your body to use. Great system design! Fruits have no obvious character flaws. Instead of acid fruits being a problem for your body, they contribute much needed alkalizing minerals that help keep your internal pH under control. They help clean up the neighborhood.

Now let's get down to the nitty-gritty practical application. If you are looking for greater detail, you'll find it in my book *An Apple a Day*? (1996). For now, we'll list some specific foods that are acid ash-producers and some that are alkaline ash-producers. Then we'll explain how to test your urine to tell if you have been overloading your alkalizing life-support system with too much acid.

THE GOOD, THE NOT-SO-GOOD, AND THE NEUTRAL

We've talked about acid ash-producing foods and alkaline ash-producing foods. You now know that, in general, acid ash foods are high protein meat, poultry, fish, and grains. You can top off that acid menu with some nuts – chopped or whole. You also know that, in general, fruits and vegetables are alkaline ash-producing foods. But notice that both groups are generalizations. There are exceptions in both. In addition, there is a small group of neutral ash foods that leave alkaline ash but have an acidifying effect on the body. (Is nothing clear cut?) These neutral ash foods include refined sugar, corn syrup, corn oil, and olive oil.

The following lists of the alkaline ash-producing foods

and acid ash-producing foods are in alphabetical order. They aren't in "strength" order. Some foods are more acidifying or alkalizing than others. These lists will give you the information you'll need when you prepare to check your urine pH. You may be surprised at how many acid ash foods you eat every day.

SOME COMMON ALKALINE ASH FOODS
(Help to control acid in your internal environment)

Almonds
Apples
Apricots
Avocados
Bananas
Barley plant juice
Beans, dried
Beet greens
Beets
Blackberries
Broccoli
Brussels sprouts
Cabbage
Carrots
Cauliflower
Celery
Chard leaves
Cherries, sour
Cucumbers
Dates, dried
Figs, dried
Grapefruit
Grapes
Green beans
Green peas
Lemons
Lettuce
Lima beans, dried
Lima beans, green
Limes
Milk, goat*
Millet
Molasses
Mushrooms
Muskmelons
Onions
Oranges
Parsnips
Peaches
Pears
Pineapple
Potatoes, sweet
Potatoes, white
Radishes
Raisins
Raspberries
Rutabagas
Sauerkraut
Soy beans, green
Spinach, raw
Strawberries
Tangerines
Tomatoes
Watercress
Watermelon

* Recommended for infants only when mother's milk is not available

SOME COMMON ACID ASH FOODS
(Leave strong acid in your internal environment)

Bacon	Eggs	Pork
Barley grain	Flour, white	Prunes^
Beef	Flour, whole wheat	Rice, brown
Blueberries	Haddock	Rice, white
Bran,wheat	Honey	Salmon
Bran, oat	Lamb	Sardines
Bread,white	Lentils, dried	Sausage
Bread, whole wheat	Lobster	Scallops
Butter	Milk, cow's^	Shrimp
Carob	Macaroni	Spaghetti
Cheese	Oatmeal	Squash,winter
Chicken	Oysters	Sunflower seeds
Cod	Peanut butter	Turkey
Corn	Peanuts	Veal
Corned beef	Peas, dried	Walnuts
Crackers, soda	Pike	Wheat germ
Cranberries	Plums^	Yogurt
Currants		

^ These foods leave an alkaline ash but have an acidifying effect on the body.

NEUTRAL ASH FOODS THAT HAVE AN ACIDIFYING EFFECT

Corn oil	Corn syrup	Olive oil	Refined sugar

THE URINE pH CHALLENGE

The purpose of checking the pH of your urine is to evaluate how your alkaline reserve is holding up and if your ammonia backup system must take the role of key acid neutralizer.

The first step of the pH challenge is to eat only acid ash-producing foods for two days. That means lots of meat, eggs, pasta, rice, chicken, bread, peanut butter, and anything else listed on the Acid Ash Foods list. But no fruit, no fruit juice, no salad, no potato chips, no banana splits, no strawberry jam – nothing listed on the Alkaline Ash Foods list.

There's no need to check your urine pH until after you have been on a strictly acid ash diet for two days. Knowing the pH of your urine doesn't tell you how your body handles excess acid if you don't know what foods your body has been processing. The "pH challenge" taken after eating a controlled diet is different from conventional pH urine tests that focus on gathering other information.

Recall that your alkaline reserve is made up of neutralizing minerals that keep strong acid left by high-protein foods from sizzling your innards. After the acid has been neutralized, it and the minerals leave your body in your urine. Your urine holds clues to whether or not, or how seriously, your supply of alkalizing minerals has been drained. If your alkaline reserve is in good shape, even though you have eaten great quantities of high – protein foods, your urine should show evidence that alkaline minerals have been the principle acid neutralizer. The condition of your alkaline reserve depends on how much high-protein food your body has had to contend with over time.

Keep in mind that we all need protein in our diets. Protein is a building block of cells, body, and health. We need protein. We don't need *too much* protein. That's what we're talking about here – too much protein!

Your pH challenge checks your alkaline reserve's ability to handle strong acid from a lot of protein. So, to make sure it's a valid test, you need a lot of protein in your body before you check your urine. That's the challenge – to see if your alkaline reserve can still handle great quantities of acid from great quantities of acid ash foods. Your alkaline reserve is being pitted against a concentrated dose of dietary acid. No point in trying to see how well dietary acid is being neutralized if you haven't eaten much high-protein food recently. This is why it's important that you eat only foods from the Acid Ash list for two days before you check your urine pH. You are going to flood your body with excess acid ash-producing protein. You might say the pH challenge is the acid test.

BUT WAIT!!!

If you are seriously ill or have a life-threatening disease – or any major illness – do not go on a diet of high protein foods. Once more, just to make sure you get that. IF YOU ARE SERIOUSLY ILL, DO NOT EAT A LOT OF HIGH PROTEIN FOODS!!!!

Remember, the purpose of monitoring pH is to evaluate an individual's health. The health of the really sick has already been evaluated – it's not good. Those who are seriously ill already have too much acid in their systems. Putting more acid ash-producing foods in a body that's already toxic from too much acid could have disastrous results. DON'T DO IT!! If you are in the seriously ill category, don't worry about your pH at this point. Just eat brown rice and as many servings of cooked vegetables as your body can tolerate.

Back to the procedure for those who are not seriously ill.

After your two full days of gluttonous gorging on steak, hamburgers, pasta, bread, rolls, eggs, cheese, sausage, biscuits, oatmeal, chicken, seafood and any other high-protein foods you can fit in, you are ready to check your urine pH. This is done on the morning of the third day at the first voiding, preferably after you have slept for at least five hours. However, if you get up several times during the night, you may not rack up five non-stop hours of rack time. Do your pH challenge when you get up to start the day. The reason you use the first voiding of the morning is that during the night your body has been doing basic "housecleaning." The first thing in the morning you get rid of most of the remnants of the previous day's food and physiological activity.

The actual procedure is simple. Reading these directions takes longer than the pH test itself.

On the morning after your two-day protein binge, as soon as you get up and go into the bathroom, tear a two- to three-inch strip of pH test paper from the roll. You will see that there is a color chart on the pH paper dispenser. This is the chart you'll use to get your urine pH number. Now, using your two- to three-inch strip of pH paper, direct one end of the paper into the urine stream very briefly – for about a second. All you need to do is get the paper wet. The paper will respond. Then match the color of the wet pH paper with a color on the dispenser chart. Note the number designated above the matching color. Dispose of the used pH paper, and write down the pH number and the current date. Take my word for it: if you don't write down your pH score, you'll forget the number before your next urine pH check, and you want to compare the two. One of the purposes of all of this is to evaluate the progress of your health – health is a process, not a one-time thing.

That's all there is to the actual pH testing. Now comes the important part. Interpreting the results. The interpretations that follow are based on clinical results gathered over thirty years of clinical practice with thousands of patients. These interpretations may not agree with your medical doctor's interpretation and understanding of urine pH. Medical urinalysis may be directed toward different evaluations. The urine pH numbers you are interpreting are intended to help you monitor your health, not to tell you how sick you are or what disease you have.

WHAT THE NUMBERS MEAN

Your urine pH numbers are alkaline reserve indicators. The "Urine pH Results" chart on page 41 gives a synopsis of the meaning of the numbers. But a little more explanation might be helpful.

Urine pH 5.5 - 5.8

If your urine scored pH 5.5 or pH 5.8, your alkaline reserve is adequate. It's holding its own. You still have enough alkalizing minerals in your body to handle a concentrated load of dietary acid. That's good. It shows that you have enough alkaline minerals to protect your kidneys from being fried by strong acid from excess protein.

You can rejoice. But don't get smug or complacent. Maybe you did well because you're still young enough that you haven't had enough meals to make major inroads into your alkaline reserve. Maybe you aren't a big meat-eater. Maybe you just like vegetables and fruit. Whatever the reason you fared so well, you need to make sure that you continue to re-equip your alkaline supply for the future.

Although your urine pH indicates that your body can handle great gobs of protein, you don't need to press the point. If you make a habit of overloading with high protein foods, your supply of neutralizing minerals will dwindle slowly. Your alkaline reserve is adequate – now. Keep it that way. Make sure you eat enough alkaline ash foods to keep it well stocked.

Now that you know your body can handle excess dietary protein, go back to your regular diet. After a couple of days, check your first voiding urine pH again. If it registers pH 6.2 or below, you are eating too much acid ash food. You need to reduce the amount of meat, poultry, fish, cheese, and grains and increase the amount of alkaline ash vegetables and fruits. No big deal, just an adjustment in quantities. You don't need to stop eating meat or other acid producers completely. Your body can handle moderate amounts of dietary acid as long as you bolster your alkaline reserve with generous amounts of replacement minerals from vegetables and fruit.

If your regular diet follow-up pH test checks in at above pH 6.2, keep doing what you're doing. You are on the right road. You probably already eat generous amounts of vegetables, fruit, and grains, and minimal amounts of meat. If you reduce the amount of grains in your diet, your pH numbers will rise even higher. That's even better.

Keep in mind that these follow-up, regular diet urine pH numbers apply only if you scored pH 5.5 or 5.8 on the acid challenge test.

Urine pH 6.0 - 6.6

Urine pH challenge test results of 6.0 to 6.6 tell a different story. It's not "good," but it's not "horrible." This is the "warning" stage. Although it would appear that your neutralizing reserves are better equipped at pH six-something rather than pH five-something, actually, the reverse is true. Your alkaline reserve is running low. However, you still have some alkalizing minerals available.

Very briefly, it works like this: The workhorse mineral of the alkaline reserve – sodium – can weaken strong acid enough to protect your delicate internal tissue. Your alkaline reserve can neutralize moderate amounts of acid from protein. It can't handle tremendous amounts of acid from protein. But for two days, you filled your digestive system with *excess* protein. There was a lot of rather strong acid to neutralize – around pH 4.5. Consequently, if your urine pH is 6.0 or above after eating *a lot* of high protein, something besides alkalizing minerals is working on the acid to bring the numbers up that high. Your alkaline reserve supply either isn't adequate to do the job by itself, or it's just overwhelmed by the volume of acid that needs to be neutralized. So backup systems begin to contribute to the neutralizing (buffering) to get the job done.

If you are in pH 6.0 - 6.6 category, in the past few months, you may have noticed more "signs of aging." You may be stiff in the morning but loosen up as the day goes on. You may tire easily or be short tempered. Your joints and muscles may be painful, and you may be more "sickly" than you once were. These annoying symptoms are easily passed off as signs that you're getting older. In reality, you are not only getting older, you are speeding the aging process by eating too much protein. Your alkaline reserves are so low that your body has called on backup systems to help neutralize too much strong dietary acid. It's beginning to get tired no matter how old you are.

However, your health outlook can be improved rather easily. Reduce the amount of high-protein acid producing foods and increase the amount of cooked vegetables in your daily diet. Since you probably don't regularly o.d. on vegetables and fruit, you should reintroduce them to your body gradually. With a morning urine in the pH 6.0 - 6.6 range, cooked vegetables do better than raw vegetables and raw fruit. That won't always be the case. As your body becomes accustomed to handling more plant food, you'll be able to eat raw vegetables and raw fruits without suffering "dietary distress" – that's the politically correct term for "belly ache."

Urine pH 6.8 - 8.0

A high urine pH seems to indicate a vast store of alkalizing minerals at work. However, that's not the case when you've challenged your body with two days of protein overload. A urine pH score of 6.8 to 8.0 when the body is saturated with dietary acid is very significant. It indicates that your supply of available alkaline reserve is virtually zilch – gone, depleted, kaput. Your system is stressed. You may be tired most of the time, have stiff joints, sore muscles, and burning on urination. This is the natural progression after the pH 6.0 - 6.6 stage if your regular diet consists mostly of acid ash foods.

A high urine pH following the acid challenge test of acid ash foods indicates that the important emergency neutralizing backup system of ammonia is the principle neutralizer. Instead of minerals neutralizing the acid from dietary protein, ammonia is doing the job.

Ammonia is produced naturally in the body through an assortment of chemical activities in almost all cells. Ammonia is also produced in the kidneys. Ammonia is a strong alkali that can give the urine a pH as high as 8.0 or more. A strong alkali (high pH numbers) can weaken a very strong acid (low pH numbers) such as sulfuric acid. And a strong alkali such as ammonia can overwhelm the kind of acid in your body that comes from acid ash (protein) foods.

The ammonia in your body is physiological ammonia. Physiological ammonia is made in your body and useful to your body. You don't put ammonia – especially household ammonia – into your body to neutralize acid. Commercially produced household ammonia – the kind you keep under lock and key so little children can't get to it and poison themselves – is strong, dangerous stuff. Your body produces physiological ammonia in specific quantities for specific uses.

Physiological ammonia produced by the kidneys helps neutralize excess acid. When the fluid in the kidneys contains too much protein due to long-term overconsumption of high protein foods, ammonia is produced as a by-product in eliminating the excess protein. The more protein in the kidney fluid, the more ammonia is produced and the higher the pH goes. When the body is overwhelmed with acid and protein, the kidneys have a lot of acid to handle. They must generate greater quantities of ammonia to handle the greater quantities of acid and protein.

But the kidneys are nearly the end point of your digestion-elimination process. By the time fluids get in the kidneys, they should have already been neutralized by your handy-dandy alkaline reserve.

Aha! You've found the key to unlock the mysteries of (1) why you can have an alkaline urine from a body that's been saturated with acid ash food, and (2) why urine smells like ammonia. And the two go together.

Your urine pH can range from quite acid (pH 4.5) to slightly alkaline (pH 8.0+) immediately following the acid challenge. Low urine pH indicates some alkaline reserve minerals are still available. High urine pH is a warning that:

1. your alkaline reserve is shot and can't neutralize the flood of acid sufficiently before it gets in the kidneys, or
2. your body is overwhelmed with large quantities of protein by-products, so
3. ammonia is produced on the spot for last chance neutralization.

That ammonia goes out with your urine and your urine pH numbers are high. And that's why if you have an alkaline urine after eating a lot of high protein foods, you have burning on urination and/or your urine smells of ammonia. It *is* ammonia. And ammonia is your body's last ditch effort to keep your innards from being stewed by excess dietary protein. Drinking cranberry juice will help relieve the burning of urination. Cranberries are acid ash foods. In juice form, the acid of cranberries travels quickly through the digestive tract and "neutralizes" the strong alkali of ammonia. Most people think the odor of ammonia is "normal" for urine. Not so. Even in children, ammonia in the urine is crisis intervention. If your urine has an ammonia odor, you know your body is fighting excess protein. And it doesn't even need to be animal protein – just too much protein.

The urine pH of strict vegetarians can be an ammonia 8.0 just as can the urine of avid meat-eaters. Many vegetarians are heavy into grains. Their diets revolve around grains. Grains in all forms. And most grains are acid ash-producers. Most nuts are also acid ash- producers. Nuts are also big favorites of most vegetarians. And your body doesn't care whether it's fighting too much dietary acid from meat or from grains and nuts. It still goes through the same survival tactics.

So, what to do if you "flunked" the urine pH challenge?

Start to improve your diet immediately, but don't toss out all of your acid ash foods and switch cold-turkey to nothing but vegetables. Your body will let you know in a hurry that it isn't accustomed to handling a sudden surge of vegetables and fruits. Your body isn't telling you it "can't" handle a lot of fruits and vegetables. It certainly can. But you probably won't like the short-term results. You see, your body has been working for a long time in its survival mode of constantly coping with excess protein. It's programmed for protein survival. A quick, radical change in diet can magnify unpleasant symptoms you already have, and it can add a few that are new. The objective is to alkalize your body slowly but surely. Begin changing your diet immediately, but make diet changes slowly enough to let your body adapt easily. You may find it helpful to jump-start the alkalizing process with nutrition supplements.

Begin your diet change very gradually. Introduce some of the "more conservative" acid ash foods, such as brown rice, into your diet and add one serving of cooked vegetables to your daily menu for a week. After a week, you can add another serving of vegetables. Continue the add-a-vegetable-a-week routine for about six weeks. That may sound like a lot of vegetables, but you have three meals a day to work with. Stick with brown rice for a while, and ease the transition with alkalizing diet supplements.

Hold off doing another urine pH check for a week or two. Give your body a little time to adjust. If you test your urine too quickly after you have started your new eating-for-health program, you may be disappointed that dramatic results don't show up immediately. Even on an improved diet, the changes in your urine pH won't be as dramatic as you might like. In fact, the pattern of change will look as though things are going from bad to worse. When the out-of-alkaline-reserve bunch improve their diets, urine pH readings go down before they start coming up again. That's because alkalizing minerals are being replenished. As more and more vegetables and fruits supply precious alkalizing minerals, urine pH goes down as in the pH 6.0 - 6.6 scenario after the pH challenge. The alkaline minerals are doing the neutralizing, not ammonia. Alkalizing minerals aren't nearly as strong on the alkaline side as is ammonia. So a steady downward trend in urine pH is great in the short term as you travel the road to health.

Your readings should change gradually – one color change at a time. If you are truly committed to improving your diet as a major part of your pursuit of health, you will probably see a dramatic change from your original pH challenge numbers in a couple of months.

But, suppose you go through all of the alkalizing processes you can think of, but your urine pH doesn't improve the way it should? You've changed your diet, cut down on acid ash foods, and eaten mostly vegetables and fruit, but your urine pH is locked in. Does that mean that it's all a waste of time? Or does it mean that this urine pH business is all a bunch of nonsense?

"No" to both of the above. There's more to pursuing health than just eating right. Other factors besides toxicity and diet enter into how your body functions. After you've "cleaned up" your diet, if you still don't feel as well as you'd like, it's time to take another type of pH test to see if emotional stress could be leading to physical distress.

EATING WELL BUT NOT FEELING YOUR BEST

Just about everyone has the occasional "down time." They just don't "feel good" despite good eating habits. They do the vegetable bit, eat very little meat, but they just aren't up to par. They are "kind of" stiff, tire easily, get out of breath just walking up stairs. How come?

Emotional override!

Their bodies are responding to strong emotions, and these responses are overriding the benefits of their good diet. That's where checking the pH of saliva comes in. Saliva pH indicates whether or not emotions are the overriding influence on physiology.

"But doesn't that smack of 'being crazy' or 'mental illness'?" you might ask.

Not at all.

We all have stress in our lives. It goes with the territory of living. If you're alive, you're stressed. But stress itself doesn't cause health problems. The way you respond might. Some ways you react to stress are more damaging to your health than others. For most of us, the biggest health hazard of all is how we cling to past hurts and injustices we have suffered and survived. And, to make matters worse, we may not even realize we are clinging!

You see, your body responds to your feelings and emotions. The most striking example of these responses is when you are suddenly and severely frightened. Fright is emotional. Your response to fright is physical. And it's fast. In extreme fright situations, the physical response is so apparent that others can tell by looking at you that you are frightened. Emotions and body are so closely intertwined that the phrase "scared to death" may not be an exaggeration.

Most of your physical responses to emotions aren't as dramatic as those of "scared to death" fright. Your physical body responds to all of your mental activities and emotions. Worry, anxiety, hate, joy, elation, and all the rest. Emotions don't have to be strong to cause a physical response. Any emotion affects your body. And when the same emotion is played over and over again for weeks, months, and years, your body continues to be affected the same way over and over. That's exhausting. Both you and your body become exhausted. And you may not be aware that anything is amiss.

But our purpose here isn't to give an in-depth study of how and why your emotions, feelings, thoughts, and memories affect your health. That's the subject of my book *Dynamic Health*. Our purpose here is to help you determine why you are feeling tired, achy, and generally "out of sorts" even though you are eating properly. That's where saliva pH comes in.

THE UPS AND DOWNS OF SALIVA pH

Saliva pH tests can indicate if "emotional override" is keeping you from feeling your best. Saliva pH isn't any more of a diagnostic tool than urine pH. Saliva pH is a tool for evaluating whether your body is responding to internal (mental and emotional) stimuli in ways that can lead to long-term health. Saliva pH tests can also provide clues to the condition of your alkaline reserve, but urine pH monitoring does a better job of that.

The pH of your saliva dances from low to high depending on what you've put into your mouth recently. The "normal" pH of saliva is considered to be around 6.8. However, it can go much lower and much higher than that. Chew on an orange, and your saliva pH can drop like a rock. Swish a solution of water and baking soda in your mouth (although I'm not sure why you would want to do that) and your saliva pH shoots up like a rocket. The point is that your saliva pH changes instantly to handle current conditions. And that's what you are looking for when you check your saliva pH – change.

This is a two-stage check. A "before" and "after." The "before" gives you the pH of your saliva when you haven't eaten anything for a while. The "after" pH shows the response to an sudden, intense "threat" of acid. Your body responds to survive "threats" of all sorts. Acid is one of those "threats." The objective is to find out if the acid "threat" is more intense than any current emotional "threat." This is where emotional override comes in – emotional threats may override physical "threats" of a sudden "acid attack." Emotions can affect the pH of your saliva. In fact, you can have residual emotional override from long-forgotten, past emotional "threats" that can send your saliva pH as low as 5.5 or as high as 8.0.

The equipment you need for your saliva pH check includes: (1) pH paper, (2) saliva, (3) a stimulant, such as a slice of lemon or a teaspoon of lemon juice, (4) a pencil and a piece of paper to record your initial results.

You begin your saliva pH check with your saliva being as close to your personal "normal" as it is likely to get when you are up, moving about, and contending with the rigors or pleasures of the day. In order to reach your daytime "saliva equilibrium" you need a period of abstinence from food, drink, and other substances that you put into your mouth. No chewing gum, no cough drops, no peppermints, no breath spray, no cigarette smoke, no toothpaste, no mouthwash. Okay, it's been two hours. You're ready to go with the pH paper, lemon, and pencil and paper.

Tear off an inch or two of pH paper. If you are reasonably healthy and have no allergies, work up some saliva and move it toward the tip of your tongue. Without touching the paper to your lips or tongue, wet the pH paper with the saliva and match the color of the wet paper with the color chart on the dispenser. Write down the pH number corresponding to the matching color.

Next, the stimulant. Put the lemon into your mouth. For this test, you *mustn't* chew. Chewing will skew the results. Just suck on the lemon until the flavor permeates your whole mouth. Dispose of the lemon. *Swallow four times* as you tear off another inch or two of pH paper, then repeat the paper-into-the-saliva routine. Compare the color and write down the corresponding pH number.

Before we get into what the numbers mean, let's back up a bit. Recall that the testing instructions began with "If you are reasonably healthy and have no allergies, work up some saliva and move it toward the tip of your tongue." There is a reason for this "reasonably healthy and have no allergies" business. Some people are too sensitive to use the pH paper in the way just described. If you are one of these, instead of touching the paper to the saliva in your mouth, put some saliva into a clean plastic teaspoon. Have your pH paper torn off and ready so you can quickly test the pH. Test the saliva immediately. Exposure to air can change the pH of the saliva rather quickly. This is the procedure for both the "before" and "after" checks.

Now you have two pH numbers and three possibilities for change. (1) The first number may be higher than the second, (2) the first number may be lower than the second, and (3) the numbers may be the same – no change. The question is, "What does it all mean?"

CHANGING COLORS

Instead of using numbers to interpret the results of your saliva pH test, we'll simplify matters and use colors instead. The color chart has three dominant colors: yellow, green, and blue. Since the colors blend into one another, to mark the change from one color to another, we'll establish color groups at particular pH numbers. We'll say that:

Yellow	=	pH 5.5 through 6.0
Green	=	pH 6.2 through 7.0
Blue	=	pH 7.2 through 8.0

Changes in saliva pH can indicate whether or not your physiology is being dominated by your emotions despite your superlative diet. Since only three possible change patterns are possible, we'll look at what each pattern of color change may indicate about your health.

Keep in mind that the color changes in the saliva test are different from color changes in urine tests. In the saliva test, you are looking at "before" and "after" changes within minutes of your body being stimulated with a quick dose of lemon juice acid. In the urine test, you look for "before" and "after" changes following days or weeks of improved diet. We're talking here about changes in saliva pH for each "double-dip" saliva test. We don't use the interpretations that follow to compare today's test results with next week's test results.

Numbers Go Up

If your pH numbers go up, this indicates that your body can respond easily to strong stimuli (acid of the lemon). No matter what color your first number was, if it changed to a higher color, that's good. Of course, some goods are better than other goods. The best "good" is green changing to blue.

Green to Blue - Preferred response

Saliva pH that starts out green and moves up to blue is the preferred response. It's a good indication that your emotions aren't getting the best of your physiology. You handle stress well, and your alkaline reserve is adequate. Since this is the preferred response it has the shortest analysis. You are entitled to a tiny bit of smugness. Just keep up the healthy diet and attitudes and check your saliva pH occasionally to make sure you are entitled to stay smug.

Yellow to Green or Blue - Not the best "good"

A yellow reading that changes to either green or blue indicates two situations, First, your alkaline reserve is holding its own. You have enough alkalizing reserve for your saliva to be flooded with alkalizing minerals to neutralize the acid of the lemon. Second, anxiety, or similar emotion, is keeping your body "on guard" most of the time. If you are feeling less than top-notch you may be emotionally stressed and not even realize it. Very likely, you are anxious much of the time. Although improper diet isn't your main problem, make sure you are kind to your body nutritionally by eating less meat and dairy products and more fruits and vegetables.

Numbers Go Down

The acid in the lemon is a sudden "threat" to your body. Your body must defend itself. The first line of defense against this threat is to neutralize the acid with alkaline saliva. This means that if the acid is the greatest threat to survival your body is facing at the moment, your saliva pH numbers will go up because your saliva is quite alkaline. If they don't go up (they go down, or stay the same) another threat, such as anxiety or other chronic stress, is dominating your physiology.

If your "after" saliva pH numbers are lower than your "before" numbers, take this as a sign that your life and health could be better with a few changes.

Blue to Green, or Green to Yellow - Wrong Direction

Your pH results indicate that your body is moving toward exhaustion. That's really not good. The problem isn't too much dietary acid. You still have alkaline reserve minerals available; that was demonstrated by the Blue or Green "before" reading. However, your digestive system is running wide-open all the time. The problem is chronic stress. Probably worry. Low-level stress that goes on and on and on. A change in lifestyle attitudes is more important than a change in diet. However, replacing meats with brown rice, and adding more vegetables can't hurt. Saliva pH responses that go down on the pH scale can serve as a warning that you could be headed for physical problems. They also indicate that you are not "doomed" to disease and despair. Both your diet and your attitudes are under your control. You can change either or both. Taking control of the way you look at life is as important as taking control of your diet. And when you take control of these two major areas of living, you take control of your health.

Numbers Don't Change

Saliva pH "before" and "after" colors that are virtually the same are the strongest indication that emotional override is the key factor. It's time to take action. Diet is essentially good but may need to be modified slightly. Emotional habits certainly need to be re-examined and modified. You can find out more about that in my book *Dynamic Health: Using Your Own Beliefs, Thoughts and Memory to Create a Healthy Body.*

Blue - Blue - Not Desirable

Blue results before and after the lemon indicate that diet isn't a major problem. The alkaline reserve is still able to sit up and take nourishment. However, true-blues have a tendency to be worriers. Some vegetarians are world-class worriers. Among other things, they worry about the animals that are killed for meat-eaters to eat. Worriers have a problem with excess digestion – it goes on constantly, even when they haven't eaten anything. However, these people usually **do not** have indigestion problems. The negative fallout from worry and anxiety overrides the positive benefits they get from their good diets. Classic emotional override. Consequently, their bodies are headed toward exhaustion.

The need for diet adjustments must be evaluated according to eating habits. Many vegetarians fall into the blue-blue category. Since they eat primarily veggies and fruit, they certainly don't need to add more. But they need to include more rice cereals with their vegetables to help neutralize the effects of anxiety such as worry. A little more acid ash in their diets might tone down their pH. However, if worry is the cause of the saliva pH readings, diet alone will not improve them.

Diet is essentially a non-issue for non-vegetarians who register blue-blue. Their bodies are being stressed by their emotions. Acute anxiety is the major problem for all blue-bluers.

Green - Green - Less Desirable than Blue - Blue

The steady-state green group is also combating emotional override. These are the "strong emotions" folks. Not only is anxiety a fixture, fear, anger, or rage are constant companions in one form or another. The end result is physical and physiological exhaustion.

Their saliva pH didn't respond to a sharp jolt of acid from the lemon. Their pH is high enough to indicate that some minerals are still available from their alkaline reserve, but the reserve isn't overflowing. They need to make a substantial change in their diet to reinforce their reserves. Less meat, more cooked vegetables, and some fruit are in order.

Their biggest challenge will be to change their long-standing negative attitudes to allow their bodies to rest occasionally. As it is, their bodies are working full-time to keep them ready day and night to fight or run. Green- green is not a good situation. Green-greeners make up much of the "physically and emotionally drained" set.

Yellow - Yellow - Serious Problems

Most people who are seriously ill are yellow-yellows. But not all people who are yellow-yellow are seriously ill. However, regardless of their present state of health, their diets and their attitudes need to be restructured immediately. Their alkaline reserve is either very low or, more likely, they are experiencing the effects of severe emotional override from persistent strong emotions such as hate, anger, or rage that they may not consciously think about. Reading *Dynamic Health* is an absolute must for yellow-yellows.

Cooked vegetables need to be added to the daily diet of yellow-yellows. The vegetables must be cooked because yellow-yellow bodies aren't ready to handle raw. Even fruit may be a bit too "strong" for their overworked systems. Changes in diet should be made gradually.

Yellow-yellows are essentially up-tight. These are the folks who need pills at night to go to sleep and coffee in the morning to get going. They may think they relax when they sleep. But they are as tired when they get up as they were when they went to bed. They may sleep, but their bodies never rest. Sorting out their emotional lives and their nutritional lives should be top priority in their daily lives if they intend to continue to have a life.

REACH YOUR POTENTIAL FOR HEALTH.

So there you have it. The rousing story of pH. Monitoring urine pH can help you to improve your menu selections. Improving your menu selections can help improve your health. But nutrition isn't the whole ball game. Monitoring saliva pH can help you determine if emotional override is heavily involved in your overall picture of health. Yet there's little point in monitoring either urine pH or saliva pH if you don't act on the information. That's the purpose behind pH monitoring and this handbook – to give you information you can use in devising your own plan of action for improving your health.

Your body's potential for health is built-in. The potential is there. Only you can cultivate or suppress it. You have seen how the types of foods you eat require your body to respond in particular ways. Every response your body makes is required for it to survive the conditions it faces at the time. Everything your body does is perfect for the circumstances. So you can't blame "poor health," or even "good health" for that matter, on your body. Your body doesn't think and it doesn't plan for the future. It works in the here and now. It works with the materials you give it. That's the good news.

With the health perspective that everything your body is doing is absolutely correct for current conditions, you realize that you have more control over your health than you had thought. That's cause for hope! You don't need to wait for disease to strike before you "do something" about your health. You don't need to depend on someone else, like your medical doctor, to "keep you well." Health is your job, not your doctor's. Your doctor does a great job when you are seriously ill, injure yourself, or when symptoms are making your life miserable or difficult. That's what doctors do. Their job is to help relieve symptoms. And they do their jobs well.

Your doctor helps you in an emergency situation when you need help fast. So, handle the crisis. After it's over, then devise your action plan for improving your health. Your doctor focuses on treating sick bodies and "fixing" parts that "misfire." We need that expertise. However, your medical doctor probably won't share your excitement over the concept of improving your health by improving your pH. That's not his or her perspective.

Health is dynamic – ever changing. Promoting health is a way of life – not a one-time thing. When you realize that your body responds to everything you put into your mouth, eating takes on a whole new flavor. And when you realize that your body responds to your attitudes, you realize your thoughts and feelings are "things" that affect your health.

Monitoring your personal pH is a tool. It's not a self-diagnostic device. Monitoring your urine pH and saliva pH can help you take charge of your health. In the final analysis, you, and only you, can lead your life in ways that promote health or in ways that prevent health. Health isn't an accident.

SYNOPSIS OF URINE pH CHALLENGE

1. Eat only acid ash-producing foods for 2 days.
2. On third day, test urine pH of first morning voiding.
3. Compare color of wet pH paper with color chart on pH paper dispenser to determine pH value of urine.
4. Refer to Urine pH Results chart.
5. Adjust diet according to pH results.

URINE pH RESULTS
First voiding of morning
Following 2-day completely Acid Ash diet

pH Reading	5.5 - 5.8	6.0 - 6.6	6.8 - 8.0
Availability of Alkaline Reserve	Adequate	Limited	Severely Limited
Ammonia	Minimal	Moderate	Maximum
Common Physical Conditions	Occasional aches and pains. Positive attitude. Hyperactive, "Type A" personality	"Sickly" Frequent joint and muscle pain. Tire easily. Short-tempered.	Frequently ill. Chronic illness. Stiff joints. Sore muscles. Headaches. General fatigue. Usually tired. Urine has ammonia odor. Possible burning on urination.
Recommended Diet Changes	Limit acid ash foods to 30% of diet. Increase amount of fruit and cooked veg. Some raw veg. are easily tolerated.	Reduce amount of acid ash foods. Increase amount of cooked vegetables. Later, add raw fruit and vegetables.	Immediately reduce amount of acid ash foods. Add cooked veg. Drink cranberry juice to relieve urinary tract burning.

SYNOPSIS OF SALIVA pH TEST

1. Wait two hours after eating or drinking (except water) to begin test.
2. Put saliva into clean plastic spoon and immediately wet pH paper with saliva.
3. Compare color of paper with color chart on dispenser.
4. Put lemon juice into mouth. Do not Chew. Allow flavor to permeate mouth, then discard.
5. Swallow four times, then retest and compare color with color chart.

SALIVA pH RESULTS and IMPLICATIONS
Yellow = pH 5.5 - 6.0 Green = pH 6.2 - 7.0 Blue = 7.2 - 8.0

pH Numbers	Go Up		Go Down	Little or No change		
Before and After Colors	Green to Blue	Yellow to Green or Blue	Blue to Green or Green to Yellow	Blue	Green	Yellow
Implication	Preferred. Normal response	Good, but could be better	Needs improve-ment	Not desirable	Not desirable	Needs immediate improving

Possible Symptoms	Occasional illness. Rapid recovery	* (See Below)	** (See Below)	** (See Below)	* (See Below)	* (See Below)
Emotional Override	Emotions not over-whelming physiology	Anxiety. Body stressed	Chronic stress. Worry slows response	Acute anxiety. Worry, short-term stress	Fear, anger, rage, anxiety	Major stress anxiety
Diet Require-ments	70% Fruit and veg 30% Meat, grains.	Reduce acid ash foods Increase fruit & veg.	Replace some meat with brown rice. Increase veg. Some fruit.	Vegetarian: Add rice cereals Non-vegetarian 70% fruit & vegetables 30% meat, and grains.	Less meat. Add cooked vegetables and some fruit.	Gradually add cooked vegetables. No raw foods until pH change possible.

* Possible Symptoms – Some or a combination of: Elevated blood pressure, heart palpitations, dilated pupils, tight muscles, increased strength, constipation, cold sweaty palms, increased mental activity, indigestion, strong reflexes, dry mouth.

** Possible Symptoms – Some or a combination of: Increased heart rate, diarrhea, increased stomach acid (ulcer), slow reflexes, weak muscles, constricted pupils, stiff joints, sore muscles, excessive tearing and saliva.